DEAN PHILLIPS

A Journey of Service and Advocacy

ETHAN REYNOLDS

TABLE OF CONTENT

INTRODUCTION

Dean Phillips: A Journey of Service and Advocacy

In the vibrant tapestry of American politics, few figures stand out quite like Dean Phillips. From his early days in the bustling city of Minneapolis, Minnesota, to his rise as a formidable force in Congress and beyond, Phillips' journey is one defined by a relentless commitment to service, innovation, and bipartisanship.

Born into a family deeply rooted in business and community engagement, Phillips inherited not only a spirit of entrepreneurship but also a profound sense of duty to his fellow citizens. These values would shape his path as he embarked on a remarkable odyssey that would lead him from the boardrooms of corporate America to the hallowed halls of the United States Capitol.

Throughout his career, Phillips has been a champion for change, tirelessly advocating for policies that advance the common good and uplift the voices of those too often overlooked by the political establishment. From his early days as a businessman to his tenure as a congressman representing Minnesota's 3rd Congressional District, Phillips has remained steadfast in his belief that true progress can only be achieved through collaboration and compromise.

But Phillips' journey is not merely one of political triumphs and legislative victories. It is also a story of personal growth and introspection, as he grapples with the complexities of leadership and the weight of responsibility that comes with serving the public good. It is a tale of resilience in the face of adversity, as Phillips navigates the turbulent waters of American politics with grace, humility, and unwavering determination.

As we embark on this journey through the life and career of Dean Phillips, we are invited to explore the depths of his character and the significance of his contributions to our nation's history. From his groundbreaking efforts to reform campaign finance to his impassioned advocacy for healthcare reform and climate action, Phillips' legacy is one that transcends partisan divides and speaks to the enduring power of principled leadership.

Through interviews, archival research, and firsthand accounts, this book seeks to capture the essence of Dean Phillips – the man, the leader, and the visionary. It is a testament to his unwavering commitment to building a better, more inclusive America for future generations. So join us as we embark on this journey into the heart and soul of one of America's most compelling political figures.

CHAPTER 1: THE EARLY YEARS

Dean Phillips was born on January 20, 1969, in Minneapolis, Minnesota, into a family deeply rooted in the local community. His father, Artie, was the CEO of Phillips Distilling Company, a business known for its innovative spirits and commitment to quality. Dean's upbringing was shaped by the values of hard work, entrepreneurship, and community engagement that were central to his family's business.

From a young age, Dean showed a keen interest in business and innovation. He often accompanied his father to the distillery, where he learned about the production process and the importance of customer satisfaction. These early experiences instilled in him a passion for entrepreneurship and a desire to make a positive impact in his community.

Dean attended local schools in Minneapolis, where he excelled academically and demonstrated strong leadership skills. He was known for his ability to bring people together and find creative solutions to problems. These qualities would serve him well in his future endeavors.

After graduating from high school, Dean went on to attend college, where he studied business and economics. During this time, he continued to be involved in various community projects and initiatives, further developing his passion for service and advocacy. Upon graduating from college, Dean joined the family business, Phillips Distilling Company, where he worked in various roles, gaining valuable experience in business management and innovation. He also became involved in philanthropy, supporting local charities and organizations that were important to him.

Dean's experiences in the business world and his commitment to community service laid the foundation for his future political career. He saw firsthand the impact that government policies could have on businesses and communities, and he became determined to make a difference in the political arena.

In 2018, Dean decided to enter politics, running for Congress in Minnesota's 3rd Congressional District. He campaigned on a platform of bipartisanship, fiscal responsibility, and campaign finance reform, believing that these issues were critical to the future of his district and the country.

Dean's campaign was a success, and he was elected to Congress, where he quickly established himself as a leader on issues such as healthcare, campaign finance reform, and climate change. He worked tirelessly to find common ground with his colleagues across the aisle, earning a reputation as one of the most bipartisan members of Congress.

Dean's early years laid the foundation for his future career in politics, shaping his values and beliefs and preparing him to make a meaningful impact in the world. His commitment to hard work, entrepreneurship, and community engagement continues to guide him as he seeks to serve the people of Minnesota and the country.

CHAPTER 2: BUSINESS AND INNOVATION

Dean Phillips' foray into the world of business began long before his entry into politics. Born into the Phillips family, known for its iconic Phillips Distilling Company, Dean grew up surrounded by the entrepreneurial spirit. As he watched his family navigate the complexities of the business world, Dean absorbed valuable lessons about hard work, innovation, and community engagement.

After completing his education, Dean joined the family business, eager to contribute and learn. He started from the ground up, working in various roles that gave him a deep understanding of the inner workings of the company. Through these experiences, Dean developed a strong work ethic and a passion for entrepreneurship that would shape his future endeavors.

Dean's journey in business took a significant turn when he became the chairman of Talenti Gelato, a position that would not only test his skills but also broaden his perspective. Leading Talenti, known for its premium gelato and sorbet, Dean faced the challenges of a competitive market while striving to maintain the company's reputation for quality and innovation.

During his time at Talenti, Dean honed his leadership abilities, implementing strategies that drove growth and profitability. His commitment to excellence and willingness to embrace new ideas earned him respect within the industry and among his peers. Beyond the day-to-day operations, Dean's tenure at Talenti also shaped his views on economic policy. He witnessed firsthand the impact of government regulations and policies on businesses, leading him to advocate for a more business-friendly environment that fosters

innovation and growth. Dean's experiences in business laid the foundation for his later political career. His time in the private sector instilled in him a deep appreciation for the role of entrepreneurship in driving economic prosperity. It also gave him a unique perspective on the intersection of business and government, shaping his approach to policy-making and governance.

As Dean transitioned from business to politics, he carried with him the lessons and values he learned in the business world. His commitment to innovation, economic growth, and community engagement would define his political career and set him apart as a leader who understood the needs and aspirations of the people he served.

CHAPTER 3: ENTRY INTO POLITICS

In 2018, Dean Phillips embarked on a journey that would reshape his life and career: a bid for Congress in Minnesota's 3rd Congressional District. Born out of a desire to bring change and accountability to Washington, Phillips's entry into politics marked the beginning of a new chapter in his life. Phillips's decision to run for Congress was not made lightly. As a successful businessman and entrepreneur, he had already made significant contributions to his community through his family's business, Phillips Distilling Company, and his leadership at Talenti Gelato. However, Phillips felt a deep sense of duty to his country and a desire to make a difference on a larger scale.

From the outset, Phillips's campaign was characterized by its emphasis on bipartisanship, fiscal responsibility, and campaign finance reform. He recognized the growing divisiveness in American politics and sought to bridge the partisan divide by working with members of both parties to find common ground on key issues.

One of the defining moments of Phillips's campaign came during the Democratic primary, where he faced off against several other candidates vying for the party's nomination. Despite being a political newcomer, Phillips's message of pragmatic problem-solving and his commitment to putting people over politics resonated with voters across the district. Throughout the campaign, Phillips crisscrossed the district, meeting with constituents, listening to their concerns, and sharing his vision for a more inclusive and accountable government. His approachable demeanor and genuine interest in the issues facing ordinary Americans set him apart from his opponents and earned him widespread support.

As the campaign entered its final stretch, Phillips emerged as the clear frontrunner, garnering endorsements from prominent Democrats and grassroots organizations alike. On Election Day, his hard work and dedication paid off as he secured a decisive victory over the Republican incumbent, flipping the seat and sending shockwaves through the political establishment. But Phillips's journey was far from over. Upon taking office, he wasted no time getting to work on behalf of his constituents, championing legislation to address healthcare, climate change, and campaign finance reform. His bipartisan approach earned him praise from colleagues on both sides of the aisle and solidified his reputation as a rising star in the Democratic Party. Looking back on his decision to enter politics, Phillips reflected on the challenges and triumphs of his campaign with a sense of pride and humility. While the road ahead would undoubtedly be difficult, he remained steadfast in his commitment to serving the people of Minnesota and fighting for a brighter future for all Americans.

CHAPTER 4: SERVICE IN CONGRESS

Dean Phillips began his service in Congress in January 2019, representing Minnesota's 3rd Congressional District. His campaign had centered on themes of bipartisanship, fiscal responsibility, and campaign finance reform, and he carried these principles into his work in the House of Representatives.

One of Phillips' early focuses was healthcare. He advocated for improving the Affordable Care Act (ACA) rather than repealing it, emphasizing the need to protect coverage for pre-existing conditions and reduce prescription drug prices. He co-sponsored bills to lower healthcare costs and expand access to care, earning praise from both Democrats and Republicans for his pragmatic approach. Campaign finance reform was another key issue for Phillips. He was a vocal critic of the influence of money in politics and co-sponsored legislation to increase transparency and accountability in campaign finance. Phillips' own campaign refused contributions from corporate PACs, a stance that resonated with voters and further solidified his reputation as a reform-minded politician. On climate change, Phillips was a strong advocate for action to address the growing environmental crisis. He supported initiatives to invest in renewable energy, reduce carbon emissions, and protect natural resources. Phillips stressed the importance of bipartisan cooperation in tackling climate change, recognizing that the issue transcends party lines and requires a united effort.

In Congress, Phillips was known for his willingness to work across the aisle. He co-founded the Problem Solvers Caucus, a bipartisan group of lawmakers dedicated to finding common ground on key issues. Phillips' collaborative approach earned him respect from colleagues on both sides of the aisle and helped him advance legislation on a variety of fronts. One of Phillips' notable achievements was the passage of the Paycheck Protection Program Flexibility Act, which he co-sponsored in response to the COVID-19 pandemic. The bill provided additional support to small businesses and workers affected by the economic downturn, demonstrating Phillips' commitment to addressing the needs of his constituents in times of crisis.

Throughout his tenure in Congress, Phillips remained true to his principles of bipartisanship and reform. He was a voice of reason in a politically polarized environment, seeking solutions that would benefit all Americans. His service in Congress solidified his reputation as a pragmatic leader willing to put aside partisan differences for the greater good.

CHAPTER 5: PRESIDENTIAL AMBITIONS

Dean Phillips' decision to run for President in 2024 was driven by a deep-seated concern for the future of American democracy and a belief that he could offer a compelling alternative to the incumbent President Joe Biden. Phillips, who had been a vocal critic of President Donald Trump, believed that Biden's leadership was lacking and that a new approach was needed to address the challenges facing the country.

Phillips launched his presidential campaign in October 2023, positioning himself as a pragmatic centrist who could bridge the divide between Democrats and Republicans. He emphasized his track record of bipartisanship in Congress, highlighting his efforts to work across the aisle on issues such as healthcare, campaign finance reform, and climate change. One of the central themes of Phillips' campaign was the need for political reform. He argued that the current system was broken, with special interests and partisan politics preventing meaningful change. Phillips proposed a series of reforms, including campaign finance reform, electoral reform, and congressional reform, to restore faith in the political process.

Throughout his campaign, Phillips faced an uphill battle against better-known candidates, including President Biden and former President Trump. He struggled to gain traction in the polls and faced criticism from some within the Democratic Party who viewed his candidacy as a distraction from the goal of defeating Trump.

Despite these challenges, Phillips remained optimistic about his chances, believing that his message of unity and reform resonated with voters across the political spectrum. He campaigned tirelessly, crisscrossing the country to meet with voters and share his vision for the future of America. However, as the primary season progressed, it became clear that Phillips' campaign was struggling to gain momentum. He failed to win any of the early primary contests, including the crucial Iowa caucuses and New Hampshire primary, and was unable to secure the endorsements of key Democratic leaders and organizations.

In February 2024, Phillips' campaign hit a major setback when he was forced to lay off staff and scale back operations due to a lack of funding. He also faced challenges in getting his name on the ballot in several states, with some state parties submitting only Biden's name for the Democratic primary.

Despite these challenges, Phillips remained committed to his campaign, believing that he had a unique perspective to offer and a duty to serve his country. However, on March 6, 2024, Phillips announced that he was dropping out of the presidential race and endorsing President Biden.

In his announcement, Phillips expressed his support for Biden and urged Democrats to unite behind the president in the upcoming election. He acknowledged that while his campaign had fallen short, he remained committed to the principles of democracy and the belief that America could overcome its challenges through unity and cooperation. Overall, Dean Phillips' presidential campaign was a testament to his commitment to public service and his belief in the power of politics to effect positive change. While his bid for the presidency may have ended in defeat, Phillips' legacy as a bipartisan leader and champion of reform will endure.

CHAPTER 6: DECISION TO WITHDRAW

Dean Phillips' decision to withdraw from the 2024 Democratic presidential primary and endorse President Joe Biden marked a significant moment in his political career. After months of campaigning and advocating for an alternative to Biden, Phillips ultimately chose to put aside his presidential ambitions in favor of party unity and the greater goal of defeating Donald Trump or other challengers in the general election.

Phillips' announcement on March 6, 2024, came as a surprise to many, as he had been campaigning vigorously and had shown no signs of slowing down. However, his campaign had faced numerous challenges, including a lack of momentum, resources, and support from within the Democratic Party. Despite these challenges, Phillips remained committed to his vision of providing an alternative to Biden and giving voters a choice in the primary.

In his announcement, Phillips spoke candidly about his decision, acknowledging that while he had entered the race to offer an alternative to Biden, it had become clear that Biden was the party's candidate and the best opportunity to demonstrate what type of country America is and intends to be.

Phillips emphasized the importance of unity within the party and the need to focus on the larger goal of defeating Trump or other challengers in the general election. His decision to withdraw and endorse Biden was met with mixed reactions. Some praised him for putting aside his personal ambitions for the greater good of the party, while others criticized him for not staying in the race and continuing to advocate for his policies and ideas. However, Phillips remained resolute in his belief that endorsing Biden was the right decision and that it was time for Democrats to unite behind him.

In the weeks following his announcement, Phillips worked tirelessly to support Biden's campaign, appearing at events and rallies across the country to rally support for the president. He also used his platform to advocate for Democratic unity and to encourage voters to turn out in support of Biden in the general election.

Overall, Dean Phillips' decision to withdraw from the 2024 Democratic presidential primary and endorse President Joe Biden was a pivotal moment in his political career. While his presidential bid may have ended, his commitment to service and advocacy remains unwavering, and his impact on the Democratic Party and the political landscape will be felt for years to come.

CHAPTER 7: CHALLENGES AND CONTROVERSIES

Dean Phillips' political career was not without its challenges and controversies. Throughout his time in office, he faced criticism from both Democrats and Republicans, who accused him of being too moderate or too partisan, depending on the issue. Phillips' willingness to work across the aisle often put him at odds with members of his own party, who viewed his bipartisanship as a betrayal of Democratic values.

One of the most significant challenges Phillips faced was the criticism of his stance on healthcare. While he supported the Affordable Care Act and other efforts to expand access to healthcare, some Democrats accused him of not going far enough in advocating for universal healthcare. Phillips defended his position, arguing that incremental change was more achievable than sweeping reforms. Another area of contention was Phillips' support for gun control measures. As a vocal advocate for gun violence prevention, Phillips pushed for stricter gun laws, including universal background checks and a ban on assault weapons. His advocacy earned him praise from gun control advocates but drew criticism from gun rights supporters, who accused him of infringing on Second Amendment rights.

Despite these challenges, Phillips remained
steadfast in his commitment to bipartisanship and finding common ground on issues that mattered most to the American people. His ability to navigate the political landscape with grace and integrity earned him respect from colleagues on both sides of the aisle, cementing his reputation as a principled and effective leader.

CHAPTER 8: PERSONAL LIFE AND PHILANTHROPY

Outside of his political career, Dean Phillips led a rich and fulfilling personal life characterized by his commitment to family and his dedication to philanthropy. This chapter delves into the various facets of Phillips' personal life, exploring his relationships, hobbies, and philanthropic

endeavors. Dean Phillips' family played a central role in his life and served as a source of inspiration and support throughout his journey. Born and raised in Minneapolis, Minnesota, Phillips grew up in a close-knit family environment. His parents instilled in him the values of hard work, integrity, and compassion, which would shape his personal and professional endeavors.

As an adult, Phillips continued to prioritize his family, cherishing moments spent with his wife, children, and extended family members. He often spoke fondly of his family in interviews and public appearances, emphasizing the importance of maintaining a strong familial bond amidst the demands of his political career.

In addition to his family life, Dean Phillips was deeply involved in philanthropy, dedicating his time, resources, and expertise to various charitable causes. His philanthropic efforts were driven by his desire to make a positive impact on the world and create meaningful change in communities near and far. One of Phillips' passions was education, and he actively supported initiatives aimed at improving access to quality education for children and young adults. He volunteered his time as a mentor and tutor, working with students from underserved communities to help them achieve academic success and pursue their dreams.

Healthcare was another area of focus for Phillips, who believed that access to affordable and comprehensive healthcare was a fundamental human right. He donated generously to healthcare organizations and advocacy groups, advocating for policies that would expand access to healthcare coverage and improve the quality of care for all Americans. Environmental conservation was also a cause close to Phillips' heart, and he supported efforts to protect natural resources and combat climate change. He invested in renewable energy projects and conservation initiatives, working to preserve the environment for future generations.

Also his direct involvement in philanthropy, Dean Phillips used his platform as a congressman to advocate for policies that would benefit marginalized communities and address systemic inequalities. He sponsored legislation aimed at reducing poverty, advancing racial justice, and promoting economic opportunity for all Americans. Throughout his personal and philanthropic endeavors, Dean Phillips embodied the values of compassion, empathy, and generosity. His commitment to making a positive difference in the world inspired others to join him in the pursuit of social justice and equality.

As Dean Phillips' political career unfolded, his personal and philanthropic commitments remained steadfast, serving as a guiding force in his efforts to create a better, more equitable society for all.

CHAPTER 9: LEGACY AND IMPACT

Dean Phillips' legacy in politics is deeply intertwined with his commitment to bipartisanship, innovation, and service. Throughout his career, he has sought to bridge the divide between Democrats and Republicans, advocating for solutions that prioritize the needs of the American people over partisan politics. While his bid for the presidency may have ended, Phillips' impact on the Democratic Party and the political landscape will be felt for years to come. One of Phillips' most significant contributions to bipartisanship was his work on campaign finance reform. He was a vocal advocate for reducing the influence of money in politics, believing that it was essential to restoring faith in the democratic process. Phillips introduced several bills aimed at reforming campaign finance laws, including the Get Foreign Money Out of U.S. Elections Act, which sought to prevent foreign entities from influencing American elections.

In addition to his work on campaign finance reform, Phillips was also a strong supporter of innovation and entrepreneurship. He believed that the government should play a role in supporting small businesses and fostering innovation, citing his own experiences in the business world as evidence of the positive impact that entrepreneurship can have on communities. Phillips championed policies that would make it easier for small businesses to access capital and navigate the regulatory landscape, earning him praise from both sides of the aisle.

Phillips' commitment to service extended beyond his work in Congress. He was actively involved in his community, volunteering his time and resources to support local organizations and causes. Phillips' philanthropic efforts focused on issues such as education, healthcare, and the environment, reflecting his belief in the importance of giving back to the community.

Despite his many accomplishments, Phillips' presidential bid ultimately fell short. His decision to withdraw from the race and endorse President Joe Biden was a testament to his commitment to putting the needs of the country above his own ambitions. Phillips urged his supporters to unite behind Biden, believing that he was the best candidate to lead the country and defend democracy against the threat posed by former President Donald Trump.

In conclusion, Dean Phillips' legacy in politics is one of bipartisanship, innovation, and service. His commitment to finding common ground and working towards solutions that benefit all Americans has left a lasting impact on the Democratic Party and the political landscape. While his presidential bid may have ended, Phillips' influence will continue to be felt for years to come, inspiring future generations of leaders to follow in his footsteps.

CONCLUSION:

In the annals of American politics, Dean Phillips' legacy will endure as a testament to the power of principled leadership, unwavering vision, and a steadfast commitment to the values that define our nation. From his early days as a businessman to his tenure in Congress and his brief but impactful foray into the presidential arena, Phillips has left an indelible mark on the political landscape of our country. Throughout his career, Phillips has embodied the spirit of bipartisanship, working tirelessly to bridge the divide between Democrats and Republicans in pursuit of common-sense solutions to the pressing issues of our time. His efforts to reform campaign finance, expand access to healthcare, and address the existential threat of climate change have set him apart as a leader unafraid to tackle the toughest challenges facing our nation.

But perhaps Phillips' greatest legacy lies in his ability to inspire others to join him in the fight for a better future. His message of unity, progress, and opportunity has resonated with Americans from all walks of life, galvanizing a new generation of leaders to step forward and carry the torch of change.

As we reflected on Phillips' journey, we are reminded that the work of building a more perfect union is never truly finished. It requires dedication, courage, and a willingness to stand up for what is right, even in the face of adversity. Phillips has exemplified these qualities throughout his career, and his legacy will continue to inspire us all to strive for a better tomorrow. As we close the chapter on Dean Phillips' story, let us not simply remember the man, but let us carry forward the lessons he has taught us – the importance of integrity, the power of collaboration, and the belief that, together, we can build a brighter future for all Americans. Dean Phillips may be stepping out of the spotlight, but his legacy will shine on as a beacon of hope and a reminder of what is possible when we work together towards a common purpose.

Dean Phillips: A Journey of Service and Advocacy
 is not just a story about one man's journey – it is a call to action for us all to rise to the challenge of creating a more just, equitable, and inclusive society. As we look to the future, let us do so with the same spirit of optimism and determination that has defined Dean Phillips' career. For in his story, we find not just inspiration, but a roadmap for how we can all make a difference in the world.

www.ingramcontent.com/pod-product-compliance
Lightning Source LLC
Chambersburg PA
CBHW071002250726
48663CB00002B/336